SUCCESSFUL PHARMACEUTICAL SELLING

SUCCESSFUL PHARMACEUTICAL SELLING

MARTIN BISCHOFF

McGraw-Hill

New York   San Francisco   Washington, D.C.   Auckland   Bogotá
Caracas   Lisbon   London   Madrid   Mexico City   Milan
Montreal   New Delhi   San Juan   Singapore
Sydney   Tokyo   Toronto

Library of Congress Cataloging-in-Publication Data

Bischoff, Martin.
    Successful pharmaceutical selling / Martin Bischoff.
      p.   cm.
    ISBN 0–7863–1211–4
    1. Selling—Drugs. 2. Pharmaceutical industry—Management.
  I. Title.
    [DNLM: Not Acquired]
    HF5439.D75B57   1997
    615.1′068′8—dc21
    DNLM/DLC   97–15126
    for Library of Congress   CIP

McGraw-Hill

A Division of The *McGraw-Hill* Companies

1 2 3 4 5 6 7 8 9 0 IU/ IU 9 0 9 8 7

ISBN 0-7863-1211-4

Printed and bound by R.R. Donnelley & Sons Company

This publication is designed to provide accurate and authoritative
information in regard to the subject matter covered. It is sold with the
understanding that neither the author nor the publisher is engaged in
rendering legal, accounting, or other professional service. If legal
advice or other expert assistance is required, the services of a
competent professional person should be sought.

> —*From a declaration of Principles jointly adopted by a*
>   *Committee of the American Bar Association and a*
>   *Committee of Publishers.*

McGraw-Hill books are available at special quantity discounts to use
as premiums and sales promotions, or for use in corporate training
programs. For more information, please write to the Director of Sales,
McGraw-Hill, 11 West 19th Street, New York, NY 10011. Or contact
your local bookstore.

The Paladin were the twelve legendary knights of Charlemagne's court who traveled the countryside doing good deeds and accomplishing heroic feats. Your mission is really not so different.

PREFACE

It is hard to imagine that a mere half century ago infections and hypertension were readily viewed as the kiss of death. Ulcers were treated with nothing less than major surgery, and people suffering from depression were confined to institutions or viewed as perhaps being possessed by malign spirits. Parkinson's disease, diabetes, angina, and arthritis could be diagnosed but not treated. A veritable multitude of afflictions that were previously dreaded are now remedied through routine visits to a physician's office.

It is clear that the quality of life enjoyed by humankind has in no small way benefited by the great advances made by the pharmaceutical industry, and leading in the parade of accomplishments are U. S. companies. No other nation, government, or business invests more money into research and development than do pharmaceutical companies. No other company or organization can point to the success that this effort has generated. Few can point with such justifiable pride in the positive impact this investment in research and development has had on society.

Yet this situation did not arise overnight. One breakthrough discovery or new concept did not precipitately propel the industry to the forefront. It required years of painstaking and often fruitless work to move pharmaceutical companies to the position of prominence they now enjoy. And in the current environment of unforgiving competition and incredibly high risk, this position can often be a tenuous one.

Pharmaceutical sales professionals play a vital role in maintaining successful companies. Their

efforts inform healthcare professionals of new products, indications, and programs. They are on the front
lines, ensuring demand and increased specification
for products, and most importantly, generating the
vital capital needed for the development of newer
and better agents. The success of their efforts ultimately determines the success of their companies.

The hallmarks of today's armies are technology
and heavy weaponry, yet it is still the foot soldier
who must take and hold ground. In an era of in-
creasingly sophisticated warfare, the soldier must
be ever more confident, trained, and well equipped
in order to fight strategically and win. This analogy
holds true for professional sales representatives,
particularly in the pharmaceutical industry. A pharmaceutical representative must be better prepared
than ever to compete, and it is the purpose of this
book to provide that winning edge.

Martin Bischoff

ACKNOWLEDGMENTS

My wife, who throughout my career has been there cajoling, sympathizing, and helping; the Newark District, for their conscientious effort over the years and critical input on this project; the training department of Pfizer Inc.; and the many outstanding sales professionals with whom I have had the honor of working over the years. To say that it has been interesting or a pleasure does not do them justice. I would also like to thank my publisher, McGraw-Hill's Healthcare Education Group and, of course, my readers.

C O N T E N T S

PART FOUR

Static

PART FIVE

Polish

PART SIX

Conclusion

SUCCESSFUL PHARMACEUTICAL SELLING

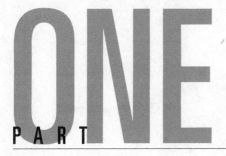

PART ONE

FRONTLINE

In the Trenches,
Making It Happen:
the Basic Elements of
Pharmaceutical Selling

There are two types of
people in this world . . .
Those with quotas. . .
and those without

Ask an experienced pharmaceutical sales representative, or a representative from any industry for that
matter, to name the core components of success
and you are likely to get as many varied answers as
the number of people who are questioned. Furthermore, the bookstores are also full of material addressing this topic. Careful analysis, however, shows
that there are really three major parts that comprise a successful pharmaceutical sales career:

- Selling skills
- Technical knowledge
- Relationships

The key here is that, like the structure of the
great pyramids, each element must balance the others and consequently form a more perfect and solid
whole. Too much emphasis on any one of
the three parts distorts the overall shape; it will not
function optimally. A harmonious blending, on the

3

other hand, replicates a design that has survived in the pyramids for millennia and serves as a constant reminder of the critical importance of equilibrium.

Certainly there have been very successful salespeople who have relied on only one or perhaps two of these components, but there are always exceptions to the rule. In order to hit the ground running and stay in the race for the entire distance, all three parts must be carefully implemented. Besides, scrutiny of a successful career will most likely reveal these three elements in any case.

All three components—selling skills, technical knowledge, and relationships—will be covered in further detail later, but each will be addressed briefly here in order to provide a framework for the detail to follow.

SELLING SKILLS

Selling skills are like the engine that drives the vehicle, the nuts and bolts that ultimately give the machine power. These are the benefits, objections, and closes that provide the framework to gain and grow business. Selling skills are the rules of the game.

There is no such thing as selling by intuition, by the seat of the pants, or from the hip—at least not for anyone who truly wants to attain success. Like any profession, set techniques and procedures must be applied and followed, and they may not be all that easy to learn and understand. Mastery of these skills cannot be avoided, however, so study them, drill them, and practice, practice, practice. The rewards are that it will get easier, and your bonuses will grow larger. Furthermore, more than one representative has commented on how these skills bring benefits in day-to-day life. Once learned, these skills are never forgotten, merely bettered!

TECHNICAL KNOWLEDGE

Most pharmaceutical representatives must attempt to barely grasp in four-plus months what it takes most physicians four-plus years, never mind the residencies, fellowships, and boards, to master. The average doctor begins practice at close to 30 years of age and well over $100,000 in debt from education loans. In other words, it takes a lot of learning to practice medicine, and please note the use of the term practice—it hasn't even been perfected!

It is into this environment that a pharmaceutical representative must not only tread, but also feel comfortable, able to compete, and ultimately win. And, just as selling skills are like an engine, technical knowledge is like the fuel and oil that it must have to run smoothly. Therefore, great emphasis must be placed on mastering the intricacies of each product; there can be no excuse for not knowing a product inside and out. Also, a solid understanding of the disease state must also be achieved. While it is impossible to acquire the same expertise as a physician, the representative must be well indoctrinated.

Technical knowledge is like running: it must be regularly exercised if you want to remain at peak form. Product and disease state knowledge must be learned and then regularly enhanced with journal reviews, training modules, and continuing education program attendance.

RELATIONSHIPS

There is no doubt that if selling skills are like an engine and technical knowledge is like the fuel and oil, then relationships are like the chrome, trim, and interior of the vehicle, all of which make the car attractive and customers willing to buy it. And, though at first glance it may seem superfluous, relationship building is as just as important as the other two sides of the pyramid.

Even the best salesperson can't sell from inside the waiting room, so getting access to the inner sanctum is essential, and it is based on knowing and working with the office staff. If two products are ultimately equal, what is the final buying decision based upon? And if just a little more business is needed to win the vice president's sales award, how is it gained?

Furthermore, pharmaceutical selling is based on long-term, repeat business. There is much more involved than merely taking an order and riding into the sunset. Not only must the products bring benefit to the physician's office, but so must the representative, personally.

And lastly, a relationship requires finesse—a human touch that distinguishes the representative as a person interested not only in his own success, but also in that of his customer. This is a quality that must be evident from the beginning and throughout a successful career in pharmaceuticals.

Components

There are many aspects of a successful sales call, from your icebreaker all the way to following up with literature and samples:

* *Icebreaker*—Your greeting must make your client comfortable and open to conversation.
* *Initial benefit statement (IBS)*—An IBS sets the stage for the presentation, and it must foster interest. It must state what your services will do for the customer.
* *Features and benefits*—You must describe a product's qualities and describe how they can help the customer.
* *Bridging*—Your presentation must move smoothly and coherently from one product to another.
* *Trial close*—You must test the water and judge the customer's response before asking for final commitment.
* *Literature*—You must leave behind clinical reports, papers, monographs, and material to support a particular point or discussion.
* *Samples*—You must allow a patient to try a product before actually filling the prescription.

The bottom line is this: a great presentation and a weak close is a weak sales call; a weak presentation but a great close equals a great sales call! Therefore, the two major components of a successful sales call are the presentation and the close. All else revolves around these key parts; without them little can be accomplished or sold.

PRESENTATIONS

There is little doubt as to the importance of a technically sound, focused, full presentation of a product. A product is sold best when it's benefits and applications can be described indepth; however, there will be occasions when a customer just does not have that much time. Nonetheless, in order to be successful, every call must result in a presentation and close.

Therefore, if you are prepared, know your stuff, have identified the doctor's needs, and are *motivated* to give a full presentation because you believe in your products, you will be successful. Yet, there are times when this might not happen—your customer may simply be too busy to see you. Those are the times to use an abridged presentation. But be cautious, for these are very limited circumstances—don't fool yourself into believing that you can get away with abridged presentations on a regular basis. Even though the doctor may want you to believe this, and the staff certainly wants you in and out, make no mistake about it: the more detail a representative can get into, the better his or her performance.

Of course, this does not mean that instead of a 10-minute presentation you can give a 20-minute one and double your sales or give a 30-minute presentation and triple your sales. It's questionable

whether a targeted customer can afford to sit around
for half an hour anyway. But what is important is de-
livering the message developed by your manager and
team at your last strategy session.

I suggest that there are three different types of
presentations:

1. *Full presentation,* as planned at district
   strategy meetings, covering all salient
   points, plenty of benefits described, and
   (hopefully) discussion and interaction with
   the physician.
2. *Semi-abridged presentation,* as may occur
   during the launch of a new product. A lot of
   time is spent presenting the new product
   and therefore other items may not be af-
   forded full coverage. Yet a major product
   can, at times, be effectively sold if the presentation developed concentrates on one
   key point (e.g., the doctor has an older
   clientele, so addressing only the renal
   safety issue might be appropriate; or if the
   practice is largely African-American, addressing only the lack of sodium retention
   in the latest study). As always, the close
   completes the representation!
3. *Abridged presentation,* for the signature-
   only situation. Again, careful analysis of
   the doctor and his or her needs and practice
   is critical. Here the goal is a feature, a benefit, and the close! This can be done in any
   situation—hospital corridor, elevator, or
   sample closet. Again, this is not the desired

approach, but it is still miles ahead of a
mere smile and query about the weather.

Again, make no mistake about it: Time spent
with the doctor translates directly into success.
Do not short-change yourself by thinking you are
gaining points with the doctor by being quick and
concise, particularly if your close competitor is giving full-blown, detailed presentations. You may be
consistently encouraged by the office staff, the doctor, and certainly your competitors to be brief.
Everybody is happy that you are heading for the
door sooner, but doing that will not get you bonuses
and promotions! You will never please everyone all
the time, and will even probably annoy a few people, but that's life and business. Whatever the situation, do your absolute best to remember the basics
of successful presentations, and good things will
surely follow!

CLOSING

Closing is, without a doubt, the single most important selling skill. This is the edge of the selling
sword, for nothing happens until the sale is closed.
It doesn't matter how good the relationship is or
how perfect the presentation unless the business
is gained. The only way to achieve this is to close
effectively.

When to close?

1. At the end of the presentation. Everything
   has been said, data presented, objections

handled and all that is left is the commitment. It is impossible to get this far and not
conclude, closing is without a doubt the logical finish.

2. The customer ends the sales call. Don't
leave the call incomplete. Ensure that something is gained: information, agreement to
continue, or better yet, some form of commitment. No better way to end a call than
with a close—what's the option—good-bye?

VIP 3. At a strong buying sign. Probably the best
time of all! Your customer is pleased and is
ready to buy—never miss this opportunity!

VIP 4. After handling an objection. Most representatives state that they are most effective
when they get into a conversation. So don't
scare the doctor off—that's why they won't
talk to us. For example, if he uses product X
don't say "well what about the associated
rash," instead try "the advantage of our
product is that it won't cause a rash."
Don't put your customer on the defensive,
product X may be his all time favorite! Be
positive and not critical, promote the advantages of your product.

Lastly, analyze the presentation itself. A technically sound and focused presentation addressing
the specific needs of a customer will lead to an easy
close. If the close is awkward or uncomfortable, then
insufficient preparation has been made. Review
your strategy, adjust the presentation, and close
again!

Types of closes

1. *The moon and stars — asking for everything!*
   Doesn't always happen but when it does the
   rewards are unforgettable. In this scenario
   the physician has committed to using your
   product for every applicable patient that
   walks in the office. This is truly the pinna-
   cle of selling and the crowning achievement
   of an outstanding product or rather because
   of an outstanding sales presentation.

2. *Increase specification and usage.* If you
   can't get it all, take just a little. Broaden
   the current prescription base by adding an
   additional indication or patient type.
   Clearly most of the time this is the close
   utilized, but over time continue this process
   and the end result may well be the moon
   and stars!

3. *In lieu of an older product or competitor.*
   Switch! Same specification but with your
   product. An excellent way to gain rapid
   acceptance particularly if there are therapeutic advantages, fewer side effects or
   lower cost.

4. *Continue what the customer is now doing.*
   Asking to do this is a commitment, of
   course, but it will not grow business. Utilize
   this only in the case where a product may
   fall out of favor or be removed from a formulary list.

Despite the importance of closing many representatives still have trouble doing it. Why is it un-

comfortable closing? If the above is followed it won't be! Close when appropriate and everyone is happy! You've earned it!

Conclusion

Key here is the fact that the presentation and, more importantly, the close drive the successful sales call. However, the more effectively all components are employed, the more effective the sales call becomes. It is no more true than here, that the sum of the parts are greater than each individually. A well-orchestrated sales call epitomizes the concept of synergy. Strive to utilize all elements, hone them to perfection, and then reap the rewards.

Pharmaceutical sales represent a unique blend of selling that is individual and separate as well as on-going and long term. No longer can one afford the luxury of viewing each sales call as a self-sustaining event. Seamless selling presents an approach to pharmaceutical sales whereby each sales technique and call becomes part of a selling continuum.

Seamless selling is an ongoing process of incremental gain, the close not being used in the traditional sense but rather to consistently expand business, unlike traditional models pictured below, which are "closed" as illustrated in Figure 1–1.

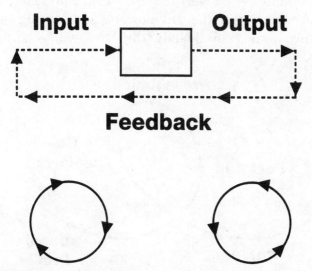

FIGURE 1–1 In the traditional sense, the closing is a cyclical, "closed" model as shown here.

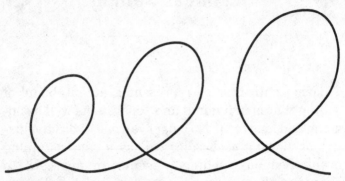

FIGURE 1–2   Seamless selling is an open, growing spiral.

Seamless selling is an open, growing spiral as depicted in Figure 1–2. Note how each component of the sales call is integrated into the expanding spiral as shown in Figure 1–3. Whether commitment is gained or not, every bit of information garnered is utilized in the preparation of the next call. The next call expands on the groundwork and intelligence gained previously. Ideally, the close will generate

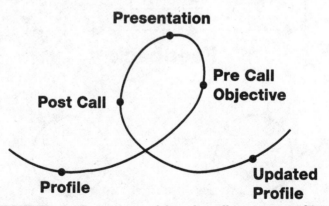

FIGURE 1–3   Components of the sales call are integrated into the expanding spiral in the seamless selling approach.

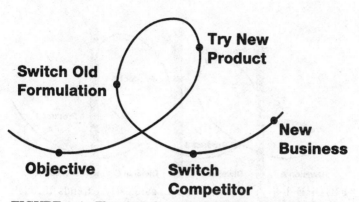

Switch Old Formulation

Try New Product

New Business

Objective

Switch Competitor

FIGURE 1–4 The expanding spiral model can be applied to a business plan and long-term strategy as well as the individual sales call.

more business; however, a failure to achieve this becomes homework for future success.

The seamless approach is also easily applied to a business plan or long-term strategy. Here, objectives are developed and refined based on the same principles used in the individual sales call. Each objective and success serves as a step toward growing business based on progress made in previous calls as illustrated in Figure 1–4.

Finally, in conjunction with teammates from other divisions, the focus is kept on coordinating efforts such that the expanding spiral seamlessly extends through divisional boundaries. Teamwork becomes the key component, as opposed to a sales technique or call as discussed above. The result again is that the continuum is unbroken and therefore fluid horizontal integration is attained.

Seamless selling attempts to impose order, direction, and a logical sequence of events, thereby

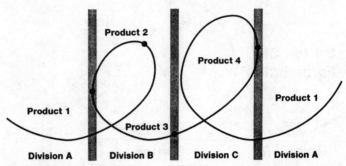

FIGURE 1–5 The spiral model seamlessly extends through divisional boundaries where teamwork then becomes the key component in expanding the spiral and growing business beyond the sales call.

providing the motivation to utilize all available tools in planning and attaining consistent sales growth. Each individual event consequently becomes part of the overall improved sales performance.

The tools presented here—physician profiles, therapeutic class reports, call objectives—whether from training, marketing, or sales administration, are all very familiar. The seamless selling technique merely provides the toolbox in which to organize them.

The Physician's Office

The Doctor's In

This is it. The center of the pharmaceutical universe. Where it all happens.

The majority of pharmaceutical products are used, and consequently promoted, in this environment. Certainly it can be daunting to anyone, even a patient, much less a professional sales representative. Unlike most selling scenarios in which the buyer goes to the seller like retail stores and car dealerships, the situation here is reversed. The seller is instead going to visit the buyer. Now as if a selling situation is not difficult enough, the buyer is clearly in his comfort zone, surrounded by his support staff and able to exert far more control than any salesperson standing behind a counter or desk.

As a result, a pharmaceutical representative must be that much better than any other kind of sales professional. He cannot rely on a manager rushing to the rescue, on high-speed demos and props, or even on the ability to walk away if the situation really deteriorates. In order to be successful here, a representative must be totally prepared mentally as well as with product knowledge, supporting documentation and a great attitude. Not so easy on a good day, never mind after waiting for an hour or two or being late due to a car accident on the interstate.

SPECIFICS

The Waiting Room

The first impression, and everyone knows just how important that is. It is here that a representative portrays himself: confident or careless, ready or reluctant. A picture is worth a thousand words but a first impression is worth far more. The office staff will often—barring those occasions when a long-time friend may enter—draw conclusions on those first critical moments when someone enters the room. Equally as important, so do patients. While a representative's time is important to the physicians, no purpose is served antagonizing their patients such that bad reports are brought back to the inner sanctum. Furthermore, a wealth of competitors' promotional literature can be found in here; spend a few moments to look around and see what is available—do not miss an opportunity to get free information.

The Front Window

Or the desk, or better yet, the front gate. There is no seeing the prescriber if this obstacle is not overcome. As will be mentioned later, no one ever sold a thing sitting in a waiting room. The staff is incredibly critical in obtaining access, information, assistance, and even a smile when things are not going so well. Spend a few moments to develop this critical resource. Remember they too have a job to do, but working together can enhance both. A warm hello, a helpful tip, or even a small box of candy can go a very long way.

The Sample Closet

An invaluable source of information, but seems of late to be getting harder and harder to access. Here is where all the patient starter samples are kept, but more importantly the prescribing habits of the healthcare providers in the office. Are the samples moving or gathering dust? Are patient education materials being handed out or deposited in the circular file? Improve your access to this resource; do not make a mess when leaving samples, maybe even tidy a bit so the staff does not sigh in exasperation upon your departure. Also do not trash your competitor's materials; not only is this the reason access to the samples is getting harder, but it is also bad business, a poor reflection of character, and even illegal.

Lastly, remember that this is an excellent place to catch a prescriber even on the busiest of days if all else fails.

The Doctor's Consult Room

The inner sanctum. If a representative is here some real selling should be about to occur. Do not ever forget, when here, the invitation is to sell. Certainly, the relationship portion of successful selling cannot be overlooked, but this is the prime opportunity to do what the profession demands. Do not squander this opportunity. Respect physicians' time; while this may also be a respite for them, nowhere is the expression "time is money" more true. Do not get too comfortable—some senior representatives have commented on the fact that they knew many of their customers since they were students, but even so, they are still a customer. Make this time count—it is becoming harder to obtain and far too precious to miss.

The Examination Room

Every so often and, unfortunately, sometimes far too often, this is where a representative may wind up waiting and selling. While certainly not ideal, it is no less an opportunity to provide a first class sales presentation. This may actually be an excellent sign demonstrating the busy schedule of the physician and the large number of patients in other rooms of the office. Be prepared, however, to make this sale standing up and perhaps using the examination table as a desk. Don't let the smell of antiseptic or the sight of syringes dissuade a great product discussion.

The Hallway

Last but not least, this locale should not be overlooked. Time for a sales presentation, no matter how exceptional, may not be in the schedule of even a semi-retired physician. Nonetheless, a brief interlude, on the way to the sample closet, checking for patient literature, or just to genuinely say hello may lend itself to an abridged presentation. Though not the most ideal situation, if the alternative is another thirty, sixty, or ninety days until the next visit, this is an excellent stopgap if even the sample closet fails!

CONCLUSION

Finally, as will be mentioned in other sections of this book, strive to make your presence an asset. Access, respect, time, and ultimately success will be all the more easily attained by being looked upon as a positive addition to the office setting. Certainly much harder to earn than perhaps suggested here, it will nonetheless pay double in the long run. It is always easier to extinguish rather than distinguish oneself, but nowhere will the benefit be as great.

Attitude

Many of the skills and techniques discussed in this book can be learned and practiced. One attribute that unfortunately cannot be picked up along the way, but rather must be there from the outset, is attitude. Attitude defines a person's feelings toward what he or she is doing. It can be negative or positive, and perhaps in many professions it really does not matter what employees' feelings are toward their day-to-day responsibilities. In sales, however, and particularly in pharmaceutical sales, attitude is everything. It is hard for a customer to get excited about a product if the individual selling it is disinterested, particularly if it is a repeat type of selling where a representative is in front of a physician every few weeks with little new to say. A positive attitude provides the stamina needed to face the stiff competition present in the industry today. And lastly, it is the stuff that differentiates mild success from great success.

Enthusiasm is a by-product of attitude. It is generated by the desire to be successful and involved in a world-leading industry, and by the knowledge that the ultimate result of your efforts is improved longevity and quality of life for many people. To be in this industry, one must want to be in it; there is little room for lukewarm interest and motivation.

Just as important as having a good attitude is showing it. Let the world know that you enjoy what you do: smile warmly, offer a welcoming handshake, and walk with pride and bearing. The greatest compliment that can be paid to you as a professional is being told that you look like you enjoy what you are doing. Truly, this is a characteristic that becomes clearly evident long before product knowledge or sales skills are mastered.

Certainly there will be periods when tough times seem to be getting the best of you: sales may be down, a major account may be lost, or personal problems may be becoming a bit overwhelming. However, this is where a good attitude really shines, because it will provide the perspective required to carry on and make it through to better days. Difficulties will ultimately pass, and a good attitude will ensure that you last.

Once in a while, take a personal inventory and acknowledge the many blessings you have. Working day-to-day sometimes makes this a bit difficult, but the results of such reflection can be amazing. We easily forget just how much we really have and should be thankful for. A quick review of the daily paper can readily illustrate this. Being involved in your local religious or charitable organization can also provide great assistance toward achieving this goal.

Ultimately, many things can be hidden with a new suit, fancy marketing materials, or a large expense account, but a bad attitude is not one of them. One's attitude is worn quite clearly, and a good one is a key ingredient in the recipe for success.

Role Playing

Just whispering these two little words can make a strong man or woman shake in terror. Nothing seems to have as unnerving an effect as the prospect of confronting peers and virtually baring one's very soul. Yet, it is the very stress and pressure caused by this exercise that makes it perhaps the most important training tool available to a representative.

A diamond is undoubtedly one of the world's most beautiful and hardest substances, yet it was once a mere lump of coal; the gem emerged only after the coal was subjected to great stress and pressure. The flawlessly executed Broadway play became so only after draining repetition, and the game-winning basket sunk only after thousands before it.

It is painfully obvious that perfection is achieved only after practice, practice, and more practice. As good as you think you are, there is always room for improvement, and rest assured that after you have mastered the game, the rules will change. As is true of professional athletes or actors, repetition and drill hone skills.

Role playing is the best way to keep at the top of your game. Every possible situation and objection can be staged, rehearsed, and refined. The role play becomes the dry run, the rehearsal of the actual selling situation. The environment can be contrived so that when it actually occurs every angle and possibility has already been reviewed. There will be no surprises.

Maximizing this training, however, requires conscious effort and the involvement of the entire sales team. Stripes must be left at the door—tenure, success, or experience cannot be used as buffers or excuses for not participating or exercising less than 110 percent.

Realistic scenarios must be employed, thus, role playing requires homework. Actual selling situations must be duplicated, customers represented, objections anticipated, and responses prepared. The role-playing scenarios practiced at the district or team level must reflect real life and go beyond the lessons of basic training. The goal is to move forward and replicate the representatives' selling environments. The purpose of role playing is to learn from mistakes when a sale is not on the line.

Utilize props or re-create a situation that caused problems in the past. Strategic practice and rehearsal make successful sales professionals.

Role plays should at a minimum be conducted in groups of three. Obviously, the salesperson and the customer must be included, but just as important is an observer. This individual becomes the key to a worthwhile exercise, carefully noting the dynamics of the scenario—what goes right and what can be done better. If he or she does the job right, the observer is actually the hardest working individual in the group.

Furthermore, role-playing sessions should be held before peers and videotaped. This allows for feedback and critical insight as to what can be improved and refined. Reviewing a videotape enables an individual to observe what actually happened. It provides a different perspective, and the chance to reconsider a given response or action and alternative courses of action. The tape can be stopped and a discussion can be initiated, a luxury unavailable during the presentation itself.

The audience, meanwhile, provides feedback and enables the all-important sharing of ideas and suggestions; this is why it is important to forget the stripes. Attacks and attitude cannot get in the way of meaningful criticism, learning, and, most importantly, praise. Furthermore, peers can see mistakes that might not get noticed by a customer but still prevent the call from being as successful as possible. On the other hand, peers also can see positives, learn from them, and benefit from the exercise.

Lastly, as in any progressive learning experience, ensure that the supervisor or manager offers some form of reward or thanks to all participants. As critical and beneficial as this is, it is nonetheless difficult and not without stress. Recognition for a job well done will provide the incentive to get in the hot seat again in the future.

Hospital Selling

Selling in hospitals or major institutions certainly incorporates different sales techniques such as more frequent use of semi- or full-abridged presentations, but underlying all of them are still the basic principles discussed throughout this book such as addressing the customer needs and closing.

Also, this section is focused at the territory level and the types of hospitals that are generally found there. Many companies have a specialized hospital or institutional representative who may be assigned to larger operations, including universities, Veterans Administration hospitals, and major medical centers. The purpose of this discussion is to merely raise the comfort level of working in the type of medium-sized hospital typically assigned to an average territory.

First and foremost, these accounts should be viewed in the same light as individual office practices, specifically what is the business potential and resulting return on investment. As many institutions are subject to formulary restrictions, active product promotion may be limited by whether or not it is approved. At a minimum, great effort and expense may have to be expended merely to achieve this status.

The most important question then, is what will be the ultimate result of having a product on formulary? If it is an office-type agent and there is no large

outpatient clinic associated with the hospital, perhaps this effort could be better focused elsewhere.
Certainly, it may be important to have formulary
status for a product merely for the prestige and example, but this should then be limited to larger and
more influential locations.

Similarly, many territories are burdened with a
fair number of hospitals, managed care organizations, long-term care facilities, and other large institutions, and it is virtually impossible to affect them
all equally. Choose carefully which of them will best
reward your efforts. Coordinate closely with company counterparts and specialists to ensure maximum coverage and influence. Most importantly, pick
your fights carefully!

When visiting facilities, moving comfortably
around these sometimes huge edifices and their
seemingly endless corridors is a necessary prerequi-
site. Spend some time acquiring maps or speaking
with security personnel to ensure that you know
where you are going. Successful hospital sales de-
pend in part on being able to find the place that will
generate the scripts; furthermore, you will en-
counter less resistance on your calls if the image you
portray is positive and confident.

Some specifics on critical areas in a hospital
include:

- *Buyer's Office*—Many institutions require
  that you stop here to sign in and pick up an
  ID badge. Though, hopefully, as time goes on,
  this may no longer be necessary, in the beginning it provides good orientation and in-

formation as to the current status of products and hospital policies.

* *CME offices*—A critical stop in any hospital call. This office can coordinate grand round speakers, displays, symposiums, and possibly even after-hours programs. Continuing Medical Education (CME) programs offer an excellent opportunity to provide third-party endorsements.

* *Pharmacy*—No doubt an absolutely key location. Certainly to gain or maintain formulary acceptance, close work with the Chief of Pharmacy or Drug Information Coordinator is essential. Furthermore, key information can be obtained as to product usage, competitor activities, in-house studies, or pending formulary changes. It is no secret that pharmacy and therapeutics (P & T) decisions are weighing more and more heavily on drug therapy utilization, and involvement and influence here is critical.

* *Department heads*—Though many department heads may not actually prescribe, their influence cannot be overlooked. Not only does the weight of their position carry significant authority, but they also may have an informal network of friends and influence gained over many years of association with the institution. Department heads may also be involved in teaching, P&T committees and selection of CME programs.

- *Outpatient clinics*—This is where most in-office products will be prescribed, although these centers may not be located directly in the hospital itself but rather off the hospital grounds nearby. Not only does this site provide an excellent opportunity to increase product specification, but also the many nurses, physician assistants, and physicians are the end users and may affect drug therapy decisions.

- *Public relations office*—An overlooked resource that can pay big returns in advertisement and relationship building. Here is where sponsorship of major campaigns, fund drives, or other such programs can be planned. Not necessarily a regular stop, but one that can prove valuable in the long run.

- *Physician's lounge*—A key location if access can be gained, but beware, this area is often verboten and usually can be entered by specific invitation only! Once inside, it is an excellent opportunity to visit with an important prescriber who may be taking a short break and looking for some diversion. However, make this stop short and pertinent, it may be the only place that many physicians may be able to really relax for a moment.

Selling in-house products such as antibiotics poses a unique situation in this environment. As is all too often the case, "selling" here may involve nothing more than a few moments in the hallway or elevator when you get a chance to hand out a two-page product monograph. This is nonetheless possible, provided such activity is not excluded by the hospital. All the more important is having these presentations perfectly tailored and focused, ensuring optimum use of the short time available.

Care must be taken, however, not to upset the flow and operations of the hospital. Many a representative has met an ill fate by not abiding by this rule—being shut out, having your products removed from the formulary, and letters of complaint sent to headquarters are only some of the consequences. Move quietly and unobtrusively, respect busy physicians and employees, and lastly, if you feel your welcome cooling, leave and come back another day.

The key here is employing the same concept as selling in an office situation: make your efforts a contribution, not a hindrance. As in the office, if the goal is to ensure the success of the account as well as your own success, then everyone will benefit and your presence will be appreciated instead of avoided.

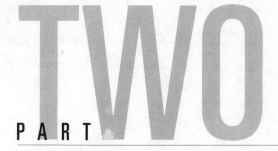

PART **TWO**

SALES SUPPORT

A Helping Hand

Resource Utilization

Pharmaceutical representatives once operated in a simpler time, an era when the factors impacting prescribing and ordering were minimal. Times, of course, have changed, and the relatively hassle-free environment of the past has given way to a system of healthcare that rivals any in its scope and complexity.

In order to survive, much less succeed in this situation, great pains must be taken to employ every possible sales support resource available. As independent as sales may seem, it is truly a complex network of interactive components all striving for the single goal of sales success. The sooner this is recognized, the sooner success will be achieved. It is, however, up to the individual to ensure that all these resources are actively engaged.

More and more companies are now employing specialty representatives highly trained in one particular area of expertise. These include managed care, federal, and national accounts, and disease-specific specialties (such as central nervous system or cardiovascular). Specialty representatives can provide valuable expertise and focus, and help to relieve already cramped schedules. By piggybacking efforts, even the most resistant customer can be assured adequate coverage and attention. Lobby aggressively to ensure that as many of these assets as possible can be dedicated to assisting in the territory.

While the lavish, all-expense-paid trips of the past may be gone, many companies still offer funding for healthcare providers to attend certain conferences. This provides an excellent opportunity not only to help obtain critical continuing education, but also to really distinguish oneself. However, these opportunities tend to be few and far between, and aggressive lobbying again may be necessary to ensure a fair share. Find out what criteria the company requires and then quickly ensure compliance—without fail.

Another valuable resource that is often neglected is medical inquiry support. Most companies provide an entire department dedicated solely to customer or representative queries. While most new representatives are intimately involved with this department, as experience grows, the use of this service declines. Yet, it provides an excellent opportunity to follow-up and provide a personal touch. Even if you know the answer, reiterating in a personalized letter that the company will provide more information can go a long way to enhancing trust and building relationships. Furthermore, sending such messages to inaccessible customers is an excellent way to ensure that some form of information is getting back to the inner sanctum. Finally, this service is often accessed electronically and is therefore simple as well as effective.

Textbooks are also outstanding door openers and thank-yous; they are also one of the last quality items the government still allows the pharmaceutical industry to distribute. These small gifts go a long way in a medical office. Healthcare providers also continue to strive to hone technical knowledge, and providing textbooks aids them greatly in achieving their goals. Many companies also still provide funding for after-hours dinner programs. These not only allow interaction with customers in a somewhat more relaxed environment, but also allow the opportunity to have a guest speaker provide third-party endorsement of a product. These events can provide an enormous return if the audience, location, and speaker are carefully selected. Any moneys provided for this activity should absolutely be maximized!

Similarly, funding may be provided to sponsor speakers at hospital lectures, grand rounds, or medical association meetings. This type of expenditure too can reap huge rewards, as third-party endorsements can reach a much larger audience in a more formal setting. Care, however, must be given to avoiding too hard a sell, as this environment is more academic and should be treated as such. Coordinate these activities with hospital continuing education departments and medical society main offices or meeting coordinators.

While the above list of resources is not all-inclusive, it does provide a firm foundation for other ideas and assets. Truly, if a representative maximizes these, greater success will be forthcoming. The key is recognizing that a territory is much like a franchise; while a representative is responsible for the ultimate success, there is considerable additional help and support available from the home office.

Time Management

The topic of time management truly has reams of books, articles, tapes, courses, and every other medium imaginable devoted to it. If there are three books on a shelf, chances are one is on time management. There are doubtless plenty of resources available if this is an area for improvement. Given the multitude of requirements facing a pharmaceutical representative today, the importance of this topic cannot be overstated. As personal time with customers diminishes, time management becomes even more important. Time in this industry is the biggest asset—and can be the most formidable enemy if it is not hoarded, managed, and maximized like any valuable resource.

Critical here, however, is first recognizing the need; like a farm, pharmaceutical sales always need something done. Work is always necessary and it consistently feels as though something is still not finished. Indeed, to be truly successful, this is the status quo.

Time management may sound simple, but keep in mind that the key to managing this resource is *determining where the business is*. Time must be spent on those customers and accounts that generate the most money. Databases should be assembled that show not only where the most business is currently achieved, but also where the most *potential* business exists. This single action is at the heart of successful territory management; it should drive all sales activity, yet is regularly overlooked.

More time, energy, and effort must be spent on the customer that can or does generate the most business—that is the painful reality. This certainly doesn't mean ignoring the little guy, but it certainly does mean balancing priorities. Waiting patiently for an hour for a target customer instead of getting immediate access to a low prescriber is certainly a worthwhile endeavor.

Institutions must be viewed in the same light. Passing on a formulary battle for gaining more retail business is not only solid time management but just plain good business. Focus on those accounts that have the most influence, dollar volume, and potential. Don't let ego get in the way of making these decisions; merely having a product on a list that generates no dollars is a hollow victory.

Also, the quantity of calls often seems to take priority over the quality of calls. This does not at all mean making one call a day, for clearly more business is achieved by making a greater number of calls. It does, however, mean ensuring that the call first results in increased product specification and second, that it is made to a high-prescribing physician. Do not be fooled into thinking that high activity alone generates sales.

Other time management techniques, such as organizing your home office, car, or day planner, can be found in any bookstore. Though not discussed here, it is, of course, very critical to success in this industry. Far more important is the weighing of the limited available resource of time, determining where it will be spent and what will be the return on investment.

Time waits for no one, but it certainly will help a competitor if it is squandered. View it as something tangible and it will be far harder to let go. Just as with finances, constantly analyze the expenditure of time and what its return yields, and that is true time management.

Teamwork—wow, what a powerful word! The number of books, articles, video and audiotapes, seminars, and programs addressing teamwork is countless. Analyze any successful individual, team, business, organization, or unit and somewhere in a big way is the aggressive implementation of teamwork.

To discuss strategies or methods enhancing or implementing this critical component is not the purpose of this book. Any library or bookstore can provide sufficient resources for addressing every approach. What is important, however, is the need to reaffirm the fact that it is key in the pharmaceutical industry as well.

A knee-jerk response might be to question the validity of teamwork as a representative goes about his daily routine without seeing coworkers for perhaps weeks at a time. Yet, it is this very fact that makes teamwork all the more important. Lacking the regular contact that an office staff or project team might have, successful teamwork is what gives the professional sales representative the winning edge.

First and foremost, synergy, or the act of combining the energy of all involved in such a way as to make it greater than that of each alone, in and of itself is positive action. Any time forces are combined and unified, effort is strengthened. The sharing of information, resources, and attitude will lead to greater individual as well as team success.

Often, work organizations are likened to sports teams in order to dramatize the mechanisms and actions of teamwork and how it can lead to championship performances. Basketball, football, and hockey leave no shortage of examples from which to draw. However, the vast majority of these teams can always win with one big play, one superstar, or one lucky break.

A far better example for this industry is a track team or cross-country running team. Anyone who has participated in these sports can immediately see the analogy. Success for the team is not predicated on one individual or event but rather on a combination of many first-, second-, and third-place finishes that result in a team victory. No one athlete can make the team win; it requires pure synergy.

Cross-country running takes the analogy one step further. A grueling, three- to five-mile run: it is won only in the long haul, not by one Herculean effort but only by the patience, determination, and guts of all the runners. Furthermore, winning scores are determined by adding the finishing places of the top five runners. It makes no difference how well the first four did; the race is not over until the fifth runner crosses the finish line.

Again, the purpose here is not to outline specific strategies or techniques, but rather to emphasize that despite the lone nature of this profession, teamwork is a vital component in the success of the company, district, and most importantly, the individ-

ual. Avoid the pitfall of deluding yourself that you
are invincible. Remember what the "team" means:

Together
Everyone
Achieves
More

Preceptorships provide an excellent avenue for developing rapport with an influential physician and learning a great deal, as well as an indirect way of influencing sales. A preceptor, or teacher, provides insight into the diagnosis and treatment of illnesses and the day-to-day operations of the practice. Consequently, students see firsthand or in essence in the field laboratory the actual application of their own and their competitors' products.

Many companies set aside funding strictly for this purpose—it is a learning experience impossible to duplicate in a corporate training center. But even if honorariums are not available, many physicians, by virtue of their pride in what they do, will agree to participate in a preceptorship. Ensure that the preceptorship is conducted with an influential and high-prescribing physician Not only will greater understanding be gained as to why physicians use certain products, but the opportunities to perhaps influence these prescribing habits are dramatically increased. Try to arrange a full-day meeting for this and attempt to assist where possible; strive to be viewed as an asset. Providing lunch on this busy day would certainly be a welcome and appropriate gesture.

Preceptorships should be conducted on a local level, and the information gained on prescribing habits should be applied to the territory. Attempt to conduct one for each product or disease state, making it a regular event if possible, but be mindful of the trade-off of making calls. Observing events such as a surgery, cardiac cath, or stress test is also an excellent extension of the concept.

Preceptorships provide an excellent vehicle for a better understanding of the daily operations of a key physician's practice. It certainly expands the knowledge and insight of the participating representative and will greatly enhance the rapport and relationship with the physician. However, it is nonetheless a support program and therefore should be used to augment, not supersede, daily sales effort. Employed as such, preceptorships will no doubt result in great returns.

Continuing Education

As previously noted, pharmaceutical representatives were once hired, trained, and, like the paladins of the past, sent on their way expecting success. Of course, every so often a new product would be introduced, and there would be a flurry of activity to learn about it and the disease state it affected. However, life seemed to revolve quite comfortably around the general rule: once trained, always trained.

Today, that rule no longer rings true. Basic training is simply that—basic training. The pharmaceutical industry, like many others relying on cutting-edge technologies, seems to change on an almost daily basis. The advances, discoveries, and new treatments that regularly appear in medical institutions and journals, trade magazines, and research facilities can be overwhelming. In the past, success meant continuous learning; now it is required to merely *compete*.

It should never be assumed that one or two learning modules on a product or disease are sufficient—this industry is far too complex for such a simplistic outlook. Many healthcare providers spend years mastering the same material to which a sales representative may dedicate a few months. After literally centuries, physicians still "practice" medicine. In this environment, a true professional must undertake a never-ending quest to continuously hone and polish technical expertise.

Fortunately, there is no end to the resources available to accomplish this goal. Certainly a good start is to begin by probing the home office training department. Many companies pride themselves on having large libraries of learning modules, tapes, and even interactive CD ROMs. Great strides are being made to offer on-line continuing education services. Get an index and get started here first.

Local institutions are also an excellent and practically required source of ongoing learning. Even the smallest community hospital will have a library with current journals and computer search capability. While a cover-to-cover analysis is not necessary, a regular review of this material surely is. Though perhaps daunting at first, this room should soon become as comfortable as your home office. Of course, get authorization to use it first.

It is critically important to read the clinicals and marketing material sent by the company. It is often frightening to observe the cavalier manner in which this material is treated. Not only will customers question the information provided, but the materials are also truly a wealth of information for the pharmaceutical representative. Ensure a solid understanding of all company-provided studies and literature and review them regularly, on your own and at local sales meetings. Almost every hospital has an ongoing continuing education program in the form of lectures, case studies, or grand rounds. Whenever possible, attend these presentations. You will not only gain a wealth of information, but have a great chance of meeting influential customers as well. Certainly, do not relent on the day-to-day business of making calls, but do realize the benefit that these programs provide in sharpening medical knowledge. Recently, many companies have offered through correspondence enrollment at the Certified Medical Representative Institute as a means of furthering education. This is an excellent means of not only enhancing your knowledge of in-line products and applicable disease states, but also of increasing your general understanding of other areas that will enhance overall professionalism and competitiveness. Inquire as to how it is possible to get involved in this most worthwhile program.

Lastly, do not overlook competitors' literature. Any form of learning can provide not only benefits, but also tremendous insights into their marketing and sales efforts. This material is always readily available in lobbies, corridors, and waiting rooms, so take advantage of it! Again, the importance of consistently honing, refining, and polishing technical expertise cannot be overstated. In an industry as dynamic as this one, a representative who seeks success cannot hope to remain static.

Computer Skills

One need not look far to see the pervasive effect of technology on society. It seems as though absolutely everything has in some way, shape, or form been computerized. Computer skills are a must in this industry. As a matter of fact, most companies have laptops at the territory level, so daily operations alone require competency in these skills.

You are virtually required to have some basic knowledge of Windows and even DOS. Most companies provide training in their own software, but learning it will be that much easier and more effective if you possess some basic knowledge. Furthermore, software today is incredibly powerful and benefits territory operations to such a great degree that it would almost be a disservice not to explore them deeper. For example:

- *On-line research*—Allows access to major medical libraries, such as the National Library of Medicine, to research literature on almost any conceivable topic. This information can be retrieved, reviewed, and printed for future reference.
- *Forecasting*—Enables projection of sales against quota and consequent analysis of what areas or accounts may require additional effort and support.
- *Graphics*—Sales in particular zip codes, accounts, or the territory as a whole can be

graphed for clear and ready review and analysis. This program may prove particularly
handy during the development of annual business plans.

+ *Word processing*—Utilized for professional-
looking invitations, thank-you notes, and co-
ordination letters. Internal reports can also
be given a far more crisp and readable edge
using any of the vast number of different
programs.

+ *Spreadsheets*—Instantly program, balance,
and monitor support program funding or any
other type of financial record keeping.

+ *Electronic mail*—Whether on the Internet or
only within the company, e-mail provides a
fast, easy method of corresponding to almost
anyone anywhere. Information can be sent
directly to accounts or offices almost instan-
taneously.

+ *CD ROM*—This medium provides a wealth
of read-only data and interactive information on compact disk. Many company training departments are now adding this tool to
their basic and home study programs.

Also available are a dizzying array of programs
allowing instant access to world news, business, and
general interest. The choice is virtually limitless,
and they can greatly aid in keeping you abreast of
current events as well as medical advances and information. Finally, in order to maximize the edge
provided by personal computers, an investment in a
typing class or two should definitely be made.

Clearly, great benefits can be gained by being even somewhat computer literate, and there is much information available on-line to be learned and shared. Several companies offer training programs in conjunction with local computer stores; if not, you may be able to get training on your own and be reimbursed. There is little doubt as to the impact computers have made in society, and certainly in this industry, using them effectively will prove invaluable.

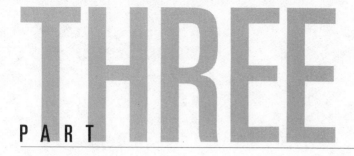

PART THREE

MAXIMIZING YOUR EFFORTS

Honing the Fine Edge

Targeting Products

Many can analyze sales...
Few can make them.

Research has shown that not only is gaining access to physicians getting more difficult, but once in the office, presentation time is also substantially shorter than years ago. It has also been suggested that the optimal number of product presentations is three, with one reminder. Consequently, what is said and in how much time is more important than ever. Time is now worth a lot more money than it was just a short time ago.

Therefore, in order to assure that what is being presented maximizes impact, extra careful analysis must be given to the prescribing habits of the practice. Exactly what products are being used and for what reasons must absolutely be determined. There once was a time when a cover-to-cover detail hitting every possible point did the trick: throw enough against the wall, and something was guaranteed to stick. Today's tougher competition and tighter schedules no longer allow for this luxury.

Many companies now provide detailed prescribing data; gone are the days of mere zip code information. Yet this data is far too often ignored, when it should in essence be a compass. Focus should be centered on what disease states are treated and with what agents. And absolutely do not waste time talking about the newest antidepressant agent if the physician and his data show he does not treat depression.

Look carefully at what diseases are being treated and, more importantly, which generate the most dollars. Clearly, pride drives us toward getting all our products presented, but ultimately that may not make the most cost-effective sales call. As with any good selling technique, go where the money is.

There is no doubt that the potential to expand business is always a possibility—that is, getting the physician to recognize and consequently treat depression—but this is not always feasible. If time is limited, then attention must be given to those products that will drive bonus dollars and rankings. Save the esoteric discussions for after-hours programs, in services, or hospital continuing education programs.

A corollary to this point is the importance of targeting the most influential healthcare professionals and those who generate the most volume. As mentioned earlier, the little guy cannot be forgotten, but to ensure solid success, focus must be on the accounts and product arenas with the greatest potential.

Learn, understand, and review the company compensation plan; it probably changes regularly. Ensure a complete understanding of what products are being emphasized, which will generate the most commission, and what will drive rankings. Make a conscious decision as to what is important, and then use that as a goal as well as a guide.

The most critical point presented in this book is the importance of targeting: targeting accounts and targeting products/disease states. This may seem somewhat callous, but in order to achieve the greatest business potential, emphasis must be placed where the results will be maximized. It is absolutely critical to work hard, but far more important to work smart.

No doubt a key component in the success of this industry is relationships. Professional sales representatives rightfully devote significant energies to developing, nurturing, and growing professional contacts.
Quite often the success of a territory or product may
very well hinge on a strong personal relationship.

Yet despite the undeniable importance of relationships, many representatives ignore the signifi-
cance of making an inward effort to be on good terms
with their immediate supervisor. A solid working relationship with a manager can result in as much of
a sales edge as one with a key customer.

Synergy results in success almost by definition.
A working situation in which there is conflict can do
nothing but detract from greater sales attainment.
No doubt that this is a two-way street, but the burden falls squarely on the shoulders of the territory
representative.

Most representatives admit they are in pharmaceutical sales because of the freedom and self-
determination the profession offers. Consequently,
demonstrate that you are truly entitled to these
opportunities—like most worthwhile things, they
must be earned. Be punctual at meetings, respond
quickly to customer's requests, work with teammates, and offer assistance to the manager whenever possible. Ask for additional work and responsibility; do not be satisfied by meeting only the

minimum requirements. Most importantly, look for things to do that will not only better your performance but also that of the team.

Be aware of the fact that even though your supervisor has your best interests at heart, there are about ten more individuals deserving attention also. But, do not forget that a manager's success depends upon the success of the territories that comprise the district or area. The suggestions, comments, and guidance are truly made to enhance performance of all concerned.

Lastly, no matter how hard we try, there are always going to be some differences with colleagues and certainly bosses. However, try to see past them and look for the greater good. Do not let quibbling and the small stuff get in the way of your bosses' and, more importantly, your own success.

❖ Managing Managed Care ❖

Even the most casual observer cannot help but notice the incredible changes that the healthcare industry has undergone in the past few years. The advent of managed care has literally revolutionized the way medicine is practiced. Consumer pressure and market forces have accomplished what government attempted and failed to do—stop the upward spiral of medical costs.

It is not the purpose of this book to debate the pros and cons of this metamorphosis; certainly numerous physicians and pharmaceutical companies have felt the pinch of evolving healthcare. A true capitalist would perhaps revel in the fact that this all occurred by virtue of supply and demand. Yet, the United States leads the world in cutting-edge technology, medical advances, and quality of medicine practiced, and this position cannot be compromised.

The bottom line is that managed care is here to stay, and we must learn to not only work within the constraints it imposes, but more importantly to thrive. The growth of managed care and international competition, and the consequent downsizing and merging of pharmaceutical organizations, have led many representatives to question the longevity of their occupation. First blush would seem to indicate that there is less and less of a call for the traditional

role of a lone salesperson calling on a solo practi-
tioner. It appears that there are more and more high-
level contracts, formularies, clinical pathways, and
group practices.

Yet, this is an industry in a state of flux, and
truly the traditional role of a pharmaceutical representative is changing. To deny this inescapable fact
is, without a doubt, to condemn the profession to ob-
solescence. However, to accept this change, embrace
it, and consequently grow with it, will lead to greater
opportunities and success.

First and foremost, product sales are always a
factor of demand. And as with the analogy of the foot
soldier in the Preface, the territory representative
must generate this. The difference now is that the
representative is no longer operating independently
with his own resources. As mentioned earlier, his
work is now a part of a spiral that includes the personnel and assets of other units that are functioning
in concert. Effort is coordinated beyond divisional
and territorial boundaries and becomes part of an
organized, *unified* operation.

This means that while managed care specialists are negotiating contracting and formulary status, line representatives are generating the interest
and enthusiasm from the healthcare providers to demand and use a given product. Neither can be successful without the other; a product cannot be utilized if it is not on formulary, and yet a product will
not be put on formulary if its advantages and benefits have not been demonstrated.

CORPORATE LEVEL

Companies as well as representatives must now also provide value-added services in addition to the product itself. This may include patient compliance and education programs, give-backs, and therapy evaluations. In the future, it will be a rare organization that focuses solely on the sales and marketing of drugs.

Of particular note here is the employment by many companies of disease management marketing efforts and programs. This concept views disease treatment as an entire package rather than just a need for pharmaceuticals. Consequently, not only does the patient benefit greatly by accessing therapies and information services previously unavailable, but so does the managed care organization by being able to share the burden of patient care.

Many organizations are also turning to some form of pharmacy benefit manager. While these operations will concentrate mostly on acquisition costs, they similarly need to be approached with contracting and value-added services. These companies will likewise need to be informed of product benefits and indications, and should be called on like any other customer.

TERRITORY LEVEL

Regularly review different plans and organizations, policies that have changed, formulary additions and deletions, and staffing changes. Analyze market data and determine which plans are making the biggest impact and move the most market share. As with any customer, use this information to strategize with counterparts as to where most resources will be applied. Concentrate on those organizations and plans that provide the best return and partnership.

Furthermore, tailor presentations according to the plan in which the customer is enrolled. Determine if minimizing time per patient, repeat visits, or cost effectiveness is the most important goal and then stress the product or support program benefit addressing this need. If available, carefully review any provider compensation plans to gather the information required to make a more focused presentation.

The careful analysis of each of the managed care organizations to which a physician may be a member is critical. This analysis should concentrate on the method of reimbursement provided by the plan. Presentations, programs, and benefits can then be customized to ensure maximum gain to the office. Consequently, in areas where managed care has a much stronger presence, representatives will have to ensure that selling strategies address the particular nuances of this high-pressure market.

GENERAL

It is readily obvious that many actions driving successful sales in the managed care arena occur at higher levels than the territory, but it is critical to ensure that *all* efforts are orchestrated and in sync with every player. Avoid the pitfall of thinking that "someone else will take care of it," or that "it ain't my job." The environment you must operate in is far too unforgiving to allow that type of attitude.

The key, however, is to also remain focused on those things that can be accomplished by the individual representative: such as providing new products or prescribing information, or samples if the organization permits them; as well as invitations to seminars, programs, and conferences; and probably most important, a much needed break during a busy day. As is true in many other businesses, success in sales is generated from a powerful ground swell—the efforts of contracting and formulary drives will mean nothing if there is no call for the product.

Working in a managed care environment can certainly appear daunting, and you may get the feeling that your individual efforts do not account for much. But remember the synergy discussion—well-coordinated individual efforts make for a very powerful punch. Act locally but plan globally, and the rewards in this arena will also be great.

Take 5!

The critical importance of nurturing and maintaining a positive, energetic attitude were discussed earlier. The demands, requirements, and quite simply the success of this profession hinge on the representative being "on" at each and every sales call. We unfortunately cannot afford the luxury of having a bad day when presenting to a customer. If you are not excited about your products, it is a sure bet your customers will not be either.

As such, the necessity to recharge one's batteries cannot be overstated. Despite the fact that each of us considers ourselves indestructible, it is simply not so. Like any other complex, finely tuned machine, we need maintenance and respite. This underscores the need to utilize vacation time and time off in order to rejuvenate. Just as the body is often called upon to fight or flight, it must also be given the opportunity to rest and repose.

Quite often, Type A personalities view this as a weakness or unproductive down time, but nothing could be further from the truth. Rest is as much of an investment in what we do as continuing education or purchasing a new PC. When one considers that we ourselves are the best sales tool, it becomes patently obvious how important our health and mental attitudes are to success.

An excellent example is getting involved in a sport hobby or some other non-work related diversion that on a regular basis provides the break discussed above. Certainly physical involvement is preferable, but any form of activity that for a short time takes you away from work will accomplish the goal. Having your family participate is all the better, providing not only impetus for taking time off but also valuable time together.

Likewise, take a coffee or lunch break during the day. These short pauses do on a daily basis what vacations and recreation do on a longer term, not only giving you that critical recharge but also affording you some time to reflect on a particular success, challenge, or course of action encountered during the workday. They offer another small investment that yields great rewards.

The key is that it is our responsibility to ensure our own well-being. Always take care of what is yours!

Addressing Needs

A critical component of successful sales of any kind is identifying a customer's "hot button." Finding and catering to this intangible quality generally garners positive results. Whether it is a textile buyer's favorite color or fabric or an office manager's preferred software package, this knowledge is essential to success. Many representatives take great pains in preparing and mastering artistic, smooth-flowing sales presentations; they are truly the Michelangelos of the industry. These presentations may be pages long and even include flowery prose. They certainly cover many aspects of the product, but do they cover what the physician wants—and, more importantly, needs—to hear?

As mentioned earlier, time is becoming more and more of a premium in today's market, thus making the few minutes available in front of a physician all the more valuable. Detailed planning and analysis must be given to a sales call in order to maximize those precious minutes. In fact, pre-call planning is as important as the actual sales call itself.

Addressing the physician's needs basically falls into two categories: personal and professional. Personal needs range from favorite sports and hobbies to preferences on how to present a product. Professional needs include type of practice, cost effectiveness of therapy, managed care constraints, and disease states treated. It makes no sense giving a first-rate presentation on angina if the physician refers all patients suffering from it to a cardiologist.

While this may sound fundamental, it is guidance rarely followed. Too often the representative becomes more engrossed in what he has to say than in what the physician wants to hear. This is also exemplified by presentations that address comparison studies with Drug X to a physician who exclusively uses Drug Y. Certainly there may be a limit to studies comparing Drug Y, but if the crossover to his reference is never made, the business is lost.

You can determine what is important to a physician from any number of sources: his staff, colleagues, or competitors, or from the doctor himself. Review prescribing data so that the presentations are to the point. Ensure that if a customer is extremely concerned about safety that efficacy is not the central theme of the presentation.

It is a worthwhile investment of time to attend seminars or read literature on different personalities and how to address them. This enables you to identify customers' preferred manner of doing business. For example, you do not want to fail to present detailed clinical data to a physician who is very analytical, or be too formal with a customer who prefers a friendly touch. Such resources help teach you to treat your clients the way *they want* to be treated—a step up from the Golden Rule.

Spending time determining and addressing a customer's needs makes solid business sense and is the foundation for success. Taking this crucial step will truly make an even and equitable playing field. Not only does this assure focused and relevant presentations, but also results in a more comfortable working relationship with the healthcare professional.

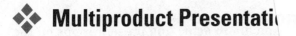

❖ Multiproduct Presentati

An ongoing challenge for any motivated sales professional is saying everything he or she wants to say during a presentation. An ideal world would allow all the time necessary to present products fully and completely, with plenty of time left for questions and answers. Unfortunately, such a world, if it ever did exist, certainly does not exist now. Not only is time sparse for a complete presentation, but it is even more so for the complete portfolio of products. Few representatives have the luxury of carrying only one product. Therefore, most representatives in the industry are challenged with regularly giving multiproduct presentations. This is no easy task by any stretch of the imagination; sometimes a coherent, technical presentation requires a lot of time, and though a physician may not have this precious resource, our responsibilities and quotas do not diminish. Creative techniques like product discussions over lunch, doughnuts, or a coffee break have always been effective and popular, but what about the rest of the day? One effective answer is to "package" presentations by using themes that carry through the entire presentation; for example, stressing a company's commitment to safety by featuring all products that do not interfere with liver function. Other themes may include once-daily dosing or unsurpassed efficacy in elderly patients. Themes consequently provide smooth bridges from product to product and aid in achieving presentations on the entire line.

Also utilize as many handouts and product reminders as possible. Often these assets are overlooked because of their simplicity, but in the course of a day any healthcare professional is bombarded with large amounts of information. Sometimes, something as simple as a pen may serve to recall an important point brought up a day or two before.

Ensure careful pre-call planning so that every word is meticulously selected to minimize time and consequently allow for as many relevant products as possible. Rambling, long-winded presentations, or too much emphasis on socializing, rarely leaves much time for more than one product. Being concise, effective, and focused will help you make the most of your time. Focus on what the doctor is actually prescribing and treating, and tailor the presentation so that every second is spent addressing his needs and practice.

Lastly, be enthusiastic! Not only is enthusiasm contagious, but it clearly wins you more time simply by its electric nature. Suddenly something special is happening, something interesting, something the physician and the staff now want to hear about. It has been said over and over that enthusiasm sells, and it certainly does, but it also gets you the time you need to make the sale.

The key here is ensuring that every effort is made to make multiproduct presentations. Do not be deluded into thinking that a second or third product can wait until the next call cycle. This can easily translate into sixty-plus days between calls! And if you see this physician only once a quarter, the interval becomes even more erosive.

Multiproduct portfolios require multiproduct presentations. Success hinges on being able to regularly present and sell the entire line. Failing to do so not only shortchanges the customer, but, more importantly, *you.*

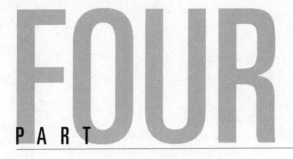

PART **FOUR**

STATIC

Fighting Interference
with the Task at Hand

Body Armor

One need not look far to realize that violent crime is on the rise in the United States. Daily we are bombarded with news that treats murder, rape, and lesser crimes as routine. Even in rural, previously safe areas crime is increasing. As a salesperson always the road, you are particularly vulnerable. A typical professional pharmaceutical representative is a well-dressed individual driving a late-model sedan; in other words, a tempting target. Furthermore, urban territories require that representatives visit areas that would be considered off limits to most other professions. It is therefore imperative that great effort be taken to secure your safe passage.

Obviously, no one wants to be the victim of a crime, much less a violent one. On a more subtle level, recovering from a crime takes time and effort that would otherwise be employed in achieving greater success—a situation that your competitor will capitalize on. Replacing stolen cell phones, PCs, and samples all takes time. Filling out police reports, repairing damage to your car, and picking up and returning rentals also consumes vast quantities of this resource. Lastly, the trials of overcoming the mental damage done by being victimized cannot be appreciated until experienced. Clearly, avoidance is the best therapy.

Reducing your profile as a target does not mean driving around in a clunker or dressing like a hobo.

It does mean, however, being slightly more aware of your surroundings and actions than the average person. Participation in defensive driving and personal safety courses is an excellent way to hone these skills. Many companies may even provide or pay for these programs if requested. The time spent at a district meeting on this issue is truly a worthwhile investment.

Jewelry, expensive watches, and accessories should be kept to a minimum. Keep PCs, phones, and other electronic gear out of sight. Minimize the amount of literature and other material in the vehicle identifying you as a representative. Keep as much material as possible in the trunk, and when possible have the necessary materials packed in your briefcase before leaving for the call; this will enable you to move immediately from the car to the office. Install a car alarm with an engine kill feature. Carry a personal alarm and try to keep one hand free for operating it (and also to quickly open doors). Try to work the rough areas in your territory in the early part of the day and avoid being there on the last day of the month.

Utilize a cell phone; they are inexpensive if used properly and invaluable in an emergency. Keep windows up and doors locked, and carry only the minimum number of credit cards and identification. Have some cash on hand so that if you are robbed you will have something to give and thereby perhaps avoid an attack.

Be aware of your surroundings; know what and who is around before accessing your trunk or doing anything that might restrict your vision. If approached by a stranger, leave immediately if possible. Minimize the time you spend in the vehicle and on the street. Lastly, if the worst event occurs and you are attacked, do not resist—equipment and samples can be replaced far easier than your health or safety.

Many of these suggestions are plain common sense, but like many well-laid plans they may be forgotten during the rush of the average workday. However, this is all the more reason to keep vigilance at its peak. In far too many reported incidents, explanations like "he came out of nowhere," or "it was only for a moment" are offered.

Again, there are numerous resources that address this topic in great depth. The intention here is merely to heighten awareness of this occupational hazard. The time spent recovering from a crime can be far better spent furthering your sales goals. In this case, more than in any other, an ounce of prevention is the path to follow.

A Question of Ethics

The healthcare community refers to prescription medications as ethical pharmaceuticals, but this does not assume that anything else is consequently unethical. Similarly, based on ongoing research, it can be safely assumed that healthcare sales representatives are also ethical. All indicators seem to consistently demonstrate that this industry is characterized by sales professionals acting in accordance with government guidelines and company policy. However, as in any industry, sport, or challenge, the white-hot heat of competition may at times blur what is right and what is not. Even without conscious decision, the moment may present itself where doing the right thing results in something less than a victory. The hallmark of a true professional is being able to recognize this and control it.

The casual omission of a potential side effect, exaggerated patient benefits, or incorrect pricing information may do more than merely damage customer relationships; ultimately, a patient may end up suffering greatly. It will only be a matter of time before the truth is realized, and whatever short-term gains may have been made will be far offset by the loss of future business. Long-term selling in the pharmaceutical industry hinges on trust; destroying that severely compromises a potentially successful career.

Recent studies suggest that ethical behavior in companies in the United States is declining. Lying to supervisors, supporting incorrect viewpoints under pressure, signing false documents, and overlooking the wrongdoing of supervisors are the major infractions. While this appears to have little to do with customer relationships, a safe assumption can be made that they are affected. Unethical conduct leads to a poor working environment, and also increases stress, reduces effectiveness, and ultimately leads to failure. The overwhelming majority of professional pharmaceutical representatives demonstrate an incredibly high level of honest, open, and ethical behavior. Yet it only takes a few bad apples to reflect poorly on the rest. Police your own ranks and dissuade any questionable behavior, but more importantly set the right example and follow only the highest standards. Rest assured that honesty is the correct course and that the benefits thereof will be realized over the course of your career.

❖ Objection/Close Notebook ❖

An objection just means someone is listening.

As discussed earlier, an objection just means someone is listening: it proves that what you are saying indeed has enough merit to warrant inquiry. An opportunity is thus provided for you to present more information and more benefits, and sell more. Furthermore, an objection is a doorway to a close.

The good news is that, believe it or not, there are only a limited number of objections that a customer can offer, and each and every one of these objections can then lead into a very specific close. Once all of these objections and closes have been identified, there should be no reason to ever miss an opportunity to ask for the business again. Make it a point to confer with teammates and assemble a notebook that lists all potential objections for a given product. Then generate responses and identify appropriate supporting material such as clinicals or monographs. For the final step, develop a close for each of these objection situations. Remember the basic rule: turn every objection into a close. Also, generate a list of closes for other situations, such as when no objection is given and the presentation is finished. Ensure that these closes refer back to the presentation and its focus. Remember, a close is earned—the weaker the preparation and presentation, the harder it is to close.

Lastly, regularly review and update this notebook. It does no good collecting dust on a bookshelf, and even the most experienced veteran can benefit. This practice may not provide us with all the answers, but should put us well on the way.

❖ Contending with Competition ❖

Sometime during your career someone is going to say, "There's enough business for everyone." Well, if that is what the competition wants to believe, great—that business is then yours. Again, there perhaps may have been a time in the past when that was true, but with today's plethora of products and international pressures, such a viewpoint is no longer valid. Business will only go to those who earn it; it will not fall like manna from Heaven.

Complicating this picture are a few individuals in government agencies who suggest that this competitive environment is forcing representatives to sell outside the prescribing information. As discussed in the ethics section earlier, the vast majority of pharmaceutical representatives are conscientious, dedicated members of the healthcare profession. Those that are successful, however, realize that a given market is of limited size and utilize all assets to maximize their product's position within it.

I am not suggesting selling directly against other agents or engaging in a mudslinging contest, but if there are studies proving your product's advantages, use them! If there are patient and cost benefits associated with your product, point them out! Ask the physician what his needs are and then demonstrate how your product fills them. And, of course after all that, close!

There are certainly going to be times when we feel more like delivery people and caterers, but that is inevitable. The key here is to utilize those techniques as a vehicle to gain selling time. Do not forget that or let the customer forget either—let the competition do that. However, when the opportunity does present itself, follow up aggressively. As mentioned earlier, time is far too precious a resource to squander.

Salespeople by nature are very sociable, often congregating and meeting with each other to share war stories, commiserate, or just hang out. These are excellent opportunities to learn what is going on from another perspective. Again, I am not suggesting fleecing a friend for information, but this is still business and as anywhere, total personal interaction is not recommended. Do not allow personal biases to interfere with your selling efforts. The fact that a family member is on a competing medication or that an old friend now works in a similar territory should not interfere with your objectives. Furthermore, do not allow any of your customers to become too close. They will always be customers and should be treated as such; otherwise, there will be less selling during presentations and it will get harder to ask for more business. And do not forget that your performance is measured by what you sell. Sales are the ultimate measure of success. No matter how well one may build relationships, relay product knowledge, or make presentations, it is the bottom line that says it all. This is the nature of the profession.

Competition is defined as a rivalry or opposition and is sometimes described as friendly, which is oxymoronic. Success in this arena is defined as growing market share—market share that another representative is also attempting to gain. One will lose it, the other have it; the former individual may as well be you! Also remember, quotas rarely decrease, and if they do, another product will make up for it. What was good enough yesterday will fall short today.

There are those in this industry who have done quite well by just chugging along, sometimes by fate, sometimes by good luck. But this does not happen all that often; to truly succeed, a representative must work hard and smart and must compete. Always play hard and play fair, but without a doubt, play to win.

Quiet Please!

Enter any elevator or common area at a hospital and it is sure to display a sign requesting quiet. It is, of course, requesting consideration for the patients being treated, but more importantly it is a small reminder to employees and staff to also respect the confidentiality of these patients. It is far too easy to discuss a particular case with a colleague, forgetting that the subject is indeed a person deserving privacy.

Similarly, our accounts and customers are people too. While at times they are often viewed as opportunities and challenges, they, like the patients discussed above, are also entitled to respect and privacy. As a result, be mindful of the manner and tone in which customers are addressed. Not only is careless discussion unprofessional, but it also may be an indicator of the way you treat this customer when actually in your presence. Professional and respectful bearing is required; it goes a long way in developing and growing solid sales relationships.

During those times when you feel you must absolutely vent your feelings, wait to do so until you are outside the building or back in your vehicle. Being overheard at these weak moments can do irreparable damage to a customer relationship. As we are all human, these flare-ups are inevitable—just pick the right time and place for them. Sometimes taking a short break can help relieve the stress.

This advice also applies quite well during company and even local sales meetings, new product launches, or conferences. Avoid making disparaging remarks about company personnel or policies; public gatherings are the absolute worst place to air gripes. While it is almost impossible to wear a smile indefinitely, these are certainly not the places to wear a frown.

Ultimately, discretion is the best guidance. Be mindful of what you say and where you say it: loose lips sank ships in World War II, and they have also torpedoed many a career. More importantly, what you say reflects on you. Ensure that this reflection is positive, professional, and finally, successful!

Access

Open, sez me.

As stated, even the world's best representative cannot sell a thing from the waiting room. To be effective, let alone successful, one must have access to the decision maker. It is always interesting to note how a representative from a smaller company with supposedly less critical products regularly gets into an important, busy office. Obviously, this individual is bringing along a little something extra. Physicians are bombarded daily with literally hundreds of commercials, messages, and presentations. Why should a physician think that yours is something special? More importantly, what differentiates you from the dozens of representatives that regularly call on that account? Furthermore, as this profession involves repeat calls and selling, how will you ensure that this access will be granted on a regular basis?

To ensure ongoing access, take care not to mistreat the office staff. Be mindful of the fact that they have jobs to do also. Respect their time as you want them to respect yours, and the payback can be great. Be courteous, friendly, and always have a ready supply of pens and notepads. And as we all know, an occasional luncheon or box of doughnuts can go a long way. Again, this may sound basic, but it is

amazing how easily such considerations can be forgotten during a typically hectic day. Always bring
along something extra—provide value-added services and you will convey the image that you are actually helping the office. Do this by promoting extra
clinicals, success stories from other customers, and
invitations to after-hours or CME programs. Always
have the required samples and ensure that your presentation is focused and tailored to the physician's
prescribing profile. Not only will this enhance your
selling efforts but it will also consequently provide
timely, interesting, and relevant information.

Strive to be viewed as a valuable asset to the
overall operation of the office. Remember, it is not
pills that we sell, but rather what they do. When a patient's hypertension is controlled, infection treated,
or ulcer healed absolutely everyone benefits. A better
selling situation cannot be achieved—be sure that
this is recognized. Your efforts consequently become
an integral part of a very important loop.

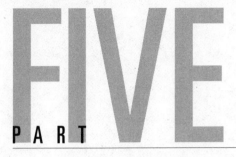

PART FIVE

POLISH

The Finishing Touches to Successful Pharmaceutical Selling

Appearance

The importance of image, how a representative carries him or herself and how he or she is perceived, was discussed earlier. Appearance is somewhat similar. Appearance is defined as the outward aspect of a person or thing. Like image, there are many books written about it—it involves a bit more than tailored garments or expensive accessories.

Once again, the importance of sharp, professional dress is not being downplayed, but to suggest that this is the only component of appearance is also wrong. Appearance embodies the individual and includes such qualities as manners and etiquette. The relationship component of pharmaceutical sales demands that a representative be able to function effectively in a social setting. Furthermore, many other personnel besides the healthcare professional are routinely encountered during the sales call. All need to be dealt with fairly, equitably and in a polite manner.

Such nuances as proper etiquette become very important due to the number of after-hours or lunch programs that many pharmaceutical representatives conduct. Learn how to properly handle silverware and maneuver through formal place settings. Maintain the same poise at the dinner table as you would in front of a desk.

Understanding and appreciation of cultural differences is also of critical importance. Learn the greetings, holidays, and dietary restrictions of the ethnic groups in the territory. Be conscious of the fact that the United States is not quite the melting pot it was years before, and cultural norms are readily practiced and displayed.

Learn a few phrases in another language. Nothing delights customers more than being able to converse, no matter how minimally, in their own tongue. A few words in a foreign language can go much farther than paragraphs of your own. Finally, watch your conversation carefully; what may have been perfectly acceptable on the last call may be totally out of place on the current one. Jokes, politics, and religion, while perhaps best avoided, are not improper but should be discussed with caution. Conversation should never be bland, but nor should it ever be abrasive.

Image should be viewed as an expression of one's internal as well as external qualities. It can reveal that there is much more than merely meets the eye—that your real virtues are more than suit- or skin-deep.

Humor

> An apple a day keeps the
> doctor away, but a smile
> sure brings 'em right back

A good sense of humor can prove to be a most valuable asset to a salesperson. It underlies a good attitude, a "stick-to-it-ive-ness" when times are tough, and a personal demeanor customers find appealing. A little humor will go a long way toward securing a rewarding career.

This is not to say that one need be a professional comedian, nor even have a sense of humor to be successful, but it does suggest that the representative who can smile and take it all in stride is ahead of the game. Being able to chuckle at life's foibles and challenges does wonders for maintaining the positive attitude required in any sales profession, much less pharmaceuticals.

Physicians by the nature of their profession see affliction and illness constantly, but rarely do people see a doctor when they are feeling well. In essence, health professionals do not necessarily see humanity when it is at its best. A representative who can offer a moment of respite during a hectic schedule, present interesting materials, and a smile provides a valuable service to the practice.

A quick word of caution: there *is* such thing as inappropriate humor. Be wary of off-color jokes and attempt to stay away from topics that border on current political correctness. As mentioned earlier, watch loose lips.

Research reveals that more facial muscles are used to frown than to smile, so for no other reason than to conserve energy needed for your next call, smile broadly. Be quick to brush off failure; grin and drive on. A little humor alone will not drive success, but it certainly will make achieving it more fun and interesting.

News

As mentioned earlier, much more goes on than what only affects business. It is critical to be involved and also aware of the myriad of current events. This not only provides a greater appreciation of life's many facets but also a better professional bearing and interesting conversation when dealing with customers.

News topics provide an excellent ice breaker before launching into a product presentation. Furthermore, this news may affect the account or customer and, consequently, business.

Newspapers are regularly full of stories of mergers, takeovers, personnel changes, and other events that affect sales. Being aware of the news permits proactive behavior and certainly fosters the appearance of being on top of things.

Every so often an article may even appear featuring a customer or immediate family member. You should always be able to readily refer to these type of interesting events. Merely clipping the article and perhaps mailing it or bringing it to the next scheduled call can start and build excellent relationships. Being well read in global affairs also sharpens impressions at company functions as well as customer-oriented affairs. Individuals interested in upward mobility can only improve their chances by moving easily from one topic of discussion to another, particularly those that affect us on a daily basis.

Often throughout this book we have seen how great gains can be made on a small investment, and it is hard to beat the return you can earn on a thirty-five-cent newspaper.

Community Involvement

Community involvement is an easy task that offers a tremendous return. Many volunteer organizations currently suggest the "fives" rule—donating 5 percent of income and five hours a week. This makes sense merely from a good citizenship perspective, giving something back to society. The benefits, however, do not stop there, for not only will the community be better, but so will business.

Practically all organizations associated with the healthcare community—the American Heart Association, the American Diabetes Association, and so on—rely on healthcare providers for programs, consultation, and leadership. Consequently, this provides an excellent, quasi-professional arena in which to make and improve business contacts, as well as free advertisement because many events are covered by local newspapers or television. How can any sales professional not benefit from positive media exposure?

Volunteer organizations such as these also provide an excellent opportunity to polish disease and product knowledge. This is a tremendous forum for gaining additional experience insight. Lacking outside influence, product knowledge can become one-dimensional and lackluster. It is a great avenue for change.

While participation in volunteer work should not be motivated solely by improving one's business standing, the positive effects on it cannot be denied. Volunteer work truly helps everyone—benefiting the community, the organization, business, and certainly oneself, so get involved and make a difference!

Promises, Promises!

> If fifty percent of people
> kept fifty percent of their
> promises fifty percent of
> the time, the world would
> be a much better place.

If 50 percent of the people kept 50 percent of their promises 50 percent of the time, the world would be a much better place. Nowhere is that more true than in a selling situation. How many times has a supervisor, colleague, or even a client promised something and then not delivered? The power of a commitment kept cannot be understated. It clearly shows that you care about yourself and, more importantly, the other person; in this case, your customer.

Everything is to be gained when we make a promise to do something and then make it happen successfully. You might even go so far as to set up a situation in which you deliberately make a commitment and then carry it out. Not only will this differentiate you as being someone who keeps your word but, even more critical, as someone who is better than the competition.

In today's fast-paced world, conversation may be fleeting, plans not refined, and agreements forgotten. The edge gained by remembering, arranging, and carrying out a promise will prove insurmountable to even the most dogged competitor.

Ultimately, a commitment becomes like a close—aggressively formulated and executed, where sales and rewards will undoubtedly follow.

A Moment of Silence

A lot can be said by saying nothing

Sometimes you can say a lot by not saying anything during a sales presentation. Often, successful salespeople are so enthusiastic about their jobs, products, and what they have to say that they do all the talking. It is a well-known fact that no one ever learned anything when they were busy talking and not listening, so then why do we do it?

The key to a successful presentation is identifying and addressing the needs and concerns of your customers, and you can only accomplish this when they can communicate them to you.

Ask probing questions and give customers time to answer; do not do it for them. Ask them how they feel and what they need, and then tell them how your products will fit into their overall scheme. And after closing, wait patiently for the response. The excitement of the sale or the fear of rejection often spurs us to provide answers to our own question. Count to five if necessary, but let the customer answer; remember we are doing the selling, not the buying!

The best sales professionals exhibit inspiration and zeal, but it is ultimately the customers who judge just how good we really are, and we will only know their opinion if we let them tell it to us!

Image

This is another topic to which reams of material have been devoted. It is a crucial component of any salesperson's success. First impressions are lasting, and in order to represent a top-notch company one must look the part. Furthermore, our customers are healthcare professionals, physicians, pharmacists, and nurses who have spent years learning their trade, and you can convey respect for them by your appearance. The importance of a professional appearance was discussed earlier and certainly cannot be understated. However, a truly professional appearance goes much deeper than that: it is the entire image that the representative presents, including clothing, grooming, and comportment.

One's demeanor is an extremely important element in successful sales or any profession. Great effort should be made to portray the picture of success we are striving to attain. Remain calm in the face of adversity and similarly when victory is at hand. Always be considerate, polite, and respectful, particularly when those around you are not. This behavior undoubtedly provides a winning edge.

The three C's are an excellent benchmark: Calm, Cool, Collected at all times. If a representative looks and acts together, access, presentations, and opinions are all enhanced. This becomes especially important when being challenged or encountering a major objection. During these situations, it is easy to crumble, show emotions, or give in, but the grace we exhibit under fire speaks volumes about our inner selves.

Above all, show no weakness. Even when dead wrong, admit it, drive on and capitalize on the opportunity that this is sure to present. At best, this could merely be a test and major victory could be within grasp. At worst, a major challenge may be about to fall, but you will be all the more ready to regroup if you are thinking clearly and are on your feet.

What is critical here is to remember that appearance addresses one's outer presentation, that is, clothing, accessories, and the like. Image is the inner component. This is the more critical stuff that demonstrates to the world what we are really made of. It is the impression that will last the longest and have the greatest impact, so ensure that it is a positive one.

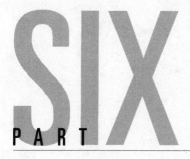

P A R T

CONCLUSION

Dare to be Different

An Anecdote

Throughout this book, I have avoided anecdotes, primarily because anyone can find some kind of story, situation, or study to support their argument. However, I will deviate this once to make my final point and conclude.

Back in grade school, we were given the popular puzzle shown below in Figure 6–1. The challenge is to connect all the dots with only four continuous lines. I took this puzzle home and worked fairly diligently on it, figuring out the answer. I found that by *folding* the paper a certain way I could indeed connect all the dots with four lines. Many classmates were stumped, for by staying within the confines of the dots it cannot be done. Only by thinking outside of the boundaries can this puzzle be solved.

The next day I strode into class feeling like King Kong. I was creative, I had the answer, and I had done it alone. Much to my chagrin, however, I found out that I was not supposed to fold the

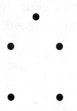

FIGURE 6–1   Connect all the dots by using four continuous lines.

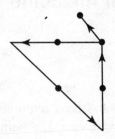

FIGURE 6–2 The solution to this puzzle requires being creative in the *right* way.

paper—that was not allowed! I was supposed to be creative, but in the *right* way (Figure 6–2).

There was an important lesson here. Even when doing an exercise that was supposed to encourage free, creative thinking there were rules. Despite the fact that I had an answer, it was different from the so-called approved solution. I thought it was merely different; instead it was just wrong.

The point is that to be successful today means stretching the conventional thinking of the past. Just because it was done one way before does not mean that it will work now. It also means going that little extra bit and being more daring and creative. Dare to try another way, shift the paradigm, break the mold, and blaze a new path. Take what is presented here, apply it in your own style, dare to be different, and you shall succeed.

ABOUT THE AUTHOR

Marty Bischoff is a 10-year veteran of pharmaceutical sales and is currently a national sales director in China for one of the globe's pre-eminent pharmaceutical companies. He has held positions in territory, hospital, and district management in several areas of the country.

His education includes a degree in Engineering from the United States Military Academy, a Masters of Public Administration from the University of Oklahoma, and he is a graduate of the Certified Medical Representative Institute. He has authored a variety of publications addressing topics in the pharmaceutical industry, U.S. military, and general interest.

This book represents a compilation of a decade's worth of experience and research into the nuances of pharmaceutical sales. Included are the observations of peers, competitors, and a healthcare environment that has radically changed over the past five years.

Marty Bischoff, a long-time resident in the cradle of the pharmaceutical industry in northern New Jersey, is currently living in Beijing, China.